THE AMERICAN HEALTH CARE CRISIS

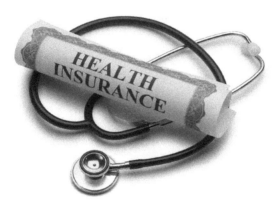

What Every American Needs to Know

Larry Stone

Copyright © 2019 Larry Stone
All rights reserved
First Edition

PAGE PUBLISHING, INC.
New York, NY

First originally published by Page Publishing, Inc. 2019

ISBN 978-1-68456-748-5 (Paperback)
ISBN 978-1-68456-750-8 (Hardcover)
ISBN 978-1-68456-749-2 (Digital)

Printed in the United States of America

Contents

I. Introduction 7
II. Brief History of Health Insurance 9
III. The Companies and Their Executives 14
IV. Litigation and Taxes 24
V. Prescription Drugs 27
VI. Potential Solutions 34
VII. A Call to Action 41
VIII. Consequences of Change 44
IX. References and Credits 47

SPECIAL THANKS

I WANT TO THANK MY lifelong friend Bill Burget. His encouragement and assistance helped make this publication possible.

I also want to thank the Center for Responsive Politics for allowing me to cite much of the information from their website, *www.opensecrets.org*.

Introduction

The problem with the high cost of health insurance and prescription drugs can be attributed to many factors with one of the primary reasons being unreasonably high profits. The industry goal of providing quality health care at the lowest price takes a back seat to their company's profits. Executives receive high salaries with their number one motivation being to increase profits for their shareholders and consequently increasing their compensation of salary and stock options. This book examines how these healthcare-related companies operate and how their way of doing business impact the cost of health insurance. Unveiled will be the unnecessary high compensation packages and other business expenses that are key factors in why Americans are paying such high premiums.

Health insurance and pharmaceutical companies operate in the marketplace like other legitimate businesses in a capitalist system. Therein lies the heart of the problem. If we are to lower the cost of health insurance and prescription drugs, we are going to have to change the way these industries operate and establish new alternative entities to make health-care costs affordable for every American. In the current system, the business practices of health-care companies completely work against the objective of low-cost health-care insurance.

Health insurance, as with other forms of insurance, is a very simple concept. A large amount of money goes into a pool out of which claims are paid. Obviously, there are many complexities. You must have actuaries to calculate risk, individuals and computers to pay claims along with a system to detect fraud. You also need a pool of individuals paying premiums in order to spread out risk. What you don't need is a Manhattan Avenue address, a very highly paid executive staff or millions of dollars spent on sales forces, marketers, lobbyists, and campaign contributions.

In the beginning, health care was provided through true nonprofit organizations. Premiums in the early plans were based solely on the cost of claims. What began as a way to provide health care for the masses morphed into one of the largest for-profit business sectors in our economy. You will also discover how the industry manipulates our politicians and is forever trying to convince the American people that they are doing their very best to provide the most affordable health-care plans possible.

America has led the world in innovation. It only makes sense that we should be able to build a better mousetrap as it relates to our current health-care system.

Brief History of
Health Insurance

Blue Cross is the basis of how the original concept of health care for the masses got its start. In the Index, you will find several books and papers used to support the research contained in these passages. They provide very interesting details as to how we got to where we are today.

In 1929, the State of Texas undertook an experiment that would forever change the health-care industry in the United States. What began as a small community project to expand health care for its residents is viewed today as a truly remarkable concept. Unfortunately, greed eventually infiltrated the original nonprofit model.

In 1929, Justin Kimball, former superintendent of Dallas Public Schools, was hired by Baylor University to consult and provide potential solutions to a rising problem. The Baylor University Hospital was struggling to pay its bills and provide care. Falling occupancy rates and the inability of patients to pay their bills had put the hospital in a dire financial situation. Justin Kimball was assigned the task of designing a plan that would help patients pay their bills, thus giving the hospital a solid financial footing. Baylor University, on the advice of Justin Kimball, designed a nonprofit plan. The plan was based on having no sales agents or middlemen and to deal directly with the hospital. Paid premiums were only to be used for hospital care for their members without any consideration for profits.

The plan became a huge success. The original plan provided twenty-one days of hospital care for $6.00 per year. In today's monetary equivalent that amounts to $96.50 per year or $8.05 per month. The plan was deemed not to be true insurance by the Texas Department of Insurance as it was viewed as a "group contract for the sale of services." Within five years of implementation, 1,300 teachers signed up for the plan along with 408 employer groups. The plan was heralded as a true way of providing affordable health care to the masses.

The original plan had only one participating hospital. But as the word of the successful Baylor plan spread across the country, individuals and states moved to improve the concept by allowing multiple hospitals to participate in these newly designed plans. It is important to note that during this era of our nation, times were extremely difficult for most Americans. Although health care was important, most Americans were struggling just to provide the necessary essentials of food and shelter for their families. Necessary health care was often delayed or totally neglected due to the inability to pay.

THE AMERICAN HEALTH CARE CRISIS

In 1931 in New Jersey, Frank Dyk, executive director of Essex County Hospital Council, was employed to oversee the collection of overdue hospital bills. He quickly realized he had an impossible task. His solution was to design a plan like the one implemented in Texas but to increase coverage by including more participating hospitals in the plan. The New Jersey plan offered twenty-one days of semi-private hospitalization for just $10 per year or less than $1 per month. Like the Baylor plan, it became a huge success and within a year six thousand people were participating along with over thirty hospitals. This is quite extraordinary considering America was in the midst of the Great Depression.

A few years later, the American Hospital Association established a goal of providing affordable health care for all members of a specific community. At the same time, they sought to give their member hospitals the financial where-with-all to survive. The success of these plans was largely due to the fact that they were nonprofit and were to be a public service supported by the community. The American Hospital Association also stipulated that their plans should not offer any financial gain to any individual or group. Initially, they elected to use the Blue Cross nonprofit model that had been so successful in areas around the nation.

The next progression of health care was the introduction of Blue Shield in 1939 that was created to reimburse medical practitioners for their services. Blue Cross and Blue Shield eventually merged in

1980 to become one entity. Today, Anthem is the largest BlueCross Blue Shield plan. They operate in fourteen states and are publicly traded on the New York Stock Exchange.

The American Hospital Association always maintained as part of their philosophy that health care was a social and civic responsibility. In the early years, marketing and enrollment were left to civic groups even including the Boy Scouts of America. Their plan design was to be free of fancy marketing materials or expensive advertising campaigns. It was simply a no-cost campaign to make members of the community aware of their options. Their goal was not a free health-care benefit but a plan that everyone could afford. The best way to accomplish that goal was to be truly nonprofit.

As our health-care options progressed past those formative years, things began to change. Large health-care insurers began to merge and began applying to state and federal regulators to change their nonprofit status. Big money came into play that included high financial returns for stockholders and large executive compensation packages. For-profit insurers quickly realized that there were vast amounts of money, ready and waiting, for their companies and shareholders. Nonprofit insurers yearned to find a way get in the game and take advantage of those same dollars. It wasn't long before profit became the number one mandate. What started out as a way for all to have affordable health care and support our medical facilities became a greed-fueled quest for profits. Most of us will agree that capitalism has played a huge role in the development of our general economy. But as you will see, health care is not something that works well within the capitalist model. Dr. James S. Todd, past executive president of the American Medical Association was quoted, "Healthy profits will become more important than healthy patients."

It is quite ironic when you consider the original purpose of devising health-care plans. By having members of the community pay a monthly affordable fee directly to the hospital, the hospital now would have the means to financially survive and in turn have the ability to provide health care to all the members of the community.

The Companies and Their Executives

Let us start out by examining the major players in the industry—their executive compensation packages and business practices. The following illustrations will show the many different factors that contribute to the high cost of health-care premiums. These examples will highlight the exorbitant compensation packages and profits in the industry of which most Americans are not aware. In quoting an often-used adage, "Just follow the money."

United Health Care

Net income for United Health Care was $10.82 billion for the year 2017.

CEO Stephen Hensley received total compensation of $15,695,513 in the year 2016.

President David Wichmann received a total compensation of $12,316,446 in the year 2016.

Larry Renfro, vice chairman and CEO of Optum received a total compensation of $12,324,995 in the year 2016.

Executive vice president and chief legal officer Marianne Short received a total compensation of $5,798,127 in the year 2016.

Executive vice president and CFO John Rex received a total compensation of $7,185,223 for the year 2016.

Humana

Humana had a net income of $1.3 billion in the year 2016.

CEO Bruce Broussard received compensation of $19,722,400 for the year 2017. This compared to an income of $8,848,066 in year 2013.

Anthem

Anthem in 2017 offered $54 billion to buy Aetna that was ultimately disapproved.

Anthem net profits were $2.47 billion for the year 2016.

CEO Joseph Swedish received compensation of $16,465,697 for the year 2016.

Angela Braley, the former CEO of WellPoint Inc., was paid $31.7 million plus $17.8 million in stock and option awards for the year 2012.

Aetna

Aetna's net income was $2.47 billion for the year 2016.

Chairman and CEO Mark Bertolini received compensation in the amount of $15 million plus $11.95 million in stock awards for the year 2014.

CFO Shawn Guertin received compensation in the amount of $3.96 million plus $2.68 million in stock and option awards for the year 2014.

Executive vice president of operations and technology Margaret McCarthy received compensation in the amount of $4.8 million plus $2.77 million in stock and option awards for the year 2014.

The executive vice president of government services received compensation in the amount of $1.48 million plus $3.38 million in stock and option awards for the year 2014.

The senior vice president of Aetna's Health and Technology Division received compensation in the amount of $7.63 million plus $5.05 million in stock and option awards for the year 2014.

Listed below are the highest 2015 compensation packages of the top 20 CEOs in the health-care industry. Information was compiled from company proxy statements, including salary, bonus, stock, and stock options. They also include any deferred compensation, perks, and other benefits.

Leonard Schleifer	Regeneron Pharmaceuticals	$47.46 million
Jeffrey Leiden	Vertex Pharmaceuticals	$28.09 million
Larry Merlo	CVS Health	$22.86 million

THE AMERICAN HEALTH CARE CRISIS

Robert Hugin	Celgene	$22.47 million
Alex Gorsky	Johnson & Johnson	$21.13 million
Michael Neidorff	Centene	$20.76 million
Alan Miller	Universal Health Services	$20.43 million
Kenneth Frazier	Merck & Co.	$19.89 million
Miles White	Abbott Laboratories	$19.89 million
John Martin	Gilead Sciences	$18.76 million
Richard Gonzalez	AbbVie	$18.53 million
Heather Bresch	Mylan	$18.16 million
David Cordani	Cigna	$17.31 million
Mark Bertolini	Aetna	$17.26 million
George Scangos	Biogen	$16.87 million
Robert Parkinson	Baxter International	$16.85 million

John Lechleiter	Eli Lilly & Co.	$16.56 million
Marc Casper	Thermo Fisher Scientific	$16.31 million
Robert Bradway	Amgen	$16.09 million
George Paz	Express Scripts Holding	$14.40 million

Lobbying

One must wonder why the health insurance industry, pharmaceutical companies, and other related health-care companies need to spend vast amounts of money lobbying our legislators. There are four health-care-related lobbyists for every congressman or congresswoman in Washington. One can be certain it is to either maintain the status quo or to change regulations for the sole purpose of increasing profits. The practice of lobbying is a way of life for businesses operating in the United States and has been for many years. Unfortunately, these lobbying expenditures equate to higher health-care premiums for all Americans.

America's Health Insurance Plans, a lobbying group for health insurance companies, spent $6,530,000 on lobbying in 2017. In the combined years of 2000 and 2001, the industry spent $21 million. The insurance industry is second in the amount of lobbying dollars compared to the drug manufacturers. This is a period in history where both industries are dedicating their lobbying efforts to change laws that are more favorable to their business practices. Not included in these figures is the huge amount of money spent to influence state insurance commissioners and legislators.

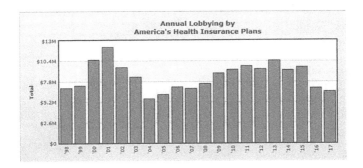

Traditionally, the largest lobbying group is the pharmaceutical/health products industry. This group includes drug manufacturers, dealers of medical products, and makers of nutritional/dietary supplements. According to the Center for Responsive Politics, these industries spent over $2.3 billion on lobbying and campaign contributions in the decade preceding 2015. Since 2005, 119 bills have come before Congress regarding the regulation of drug pricing. None of these bills ever passed. The industry is obviously getting their money's worth from their lobbying efforts.

LARRY STONE

Top recipients of health-care industry lobbyist dollars for 2017–2018

Paul Ryan (R-WI)	House	$842,899
Sherrod Brown (D-OH)	Senate	$756,870
Greg Walden (R-OR)	House	$690,000
Orin Hatch (R-UT)	Senate	$689,582
Bob Casey (D-PA)	Senate	$684,773
Jon Ossoff (D-GA)	Not Elected	$599,960
Kevin Brady (R-TX)	House	$567,050
Kevin McCarthy (R-CA)	House	$517,645
Bill Nelson (D-FL)	Senate	$451,105
John Barrasso (R-WY)	Senate	$447,425
Michael Burgess (R-TX)	House	$445,365

THE AMERICAN HEALTH CARE CRISIS

Bill Cassidy (R-LA)	Senate	$444,620
Raja Krishnamoorthi (D-IL)	House	$431,702
Debbie Stabenow (D-MI)	Senate	$405,887
Dean Heller (R-NV)	Senate	$379,659
Tammy Baldwin (D-WI)	Senate	$370,973
Kirsten Gillibrand (D-NY)	Senate	$367,345
Raul Ruiz (D-CA)	House	$362,074

Top pharmaceutical and health products political contributors for 2017–2018

Pfizer Inc.	$916,039
Amgen Inc.	$836,655
DE Shaw Research	$764,644
Express Scripts	$684,380
Health Foods of America	$651,325

Abbvie Inc.	$645,719
Amerisource Bergen Corp.	$589,566
Johnson & Johnson	$537,693
Eli Lilly & Co.	$502,371
Merck & Co.	$470,373
Stark Hearing Technologies	$465,918
Exoxemis	$455,400
Abbot Laboratories	$387,748
Ischemix	$382,000
Sanofi	$375,817
McKesson Corp.	$372,154
Genentech Inc.	$367,610
AstraZeneca PLC	$348,068
Nova Nordisk	$345,473
Celegene Corp.	$310,410

All donations took place during the 2017–2018 election cycle and were released by the Federal Election Commission on Monday, March 26, 2018.

An entire book could be written on lobbying and how lobbyists influence policy and help enact laws that are not in the best interest of the American consumer. When looking at lobbying dollars, what we don't see, is what is called the "the revolving door." This is when a legislator or staffer leaves government service and becomes a lobbyist.

When the prescription benefit Medicare Part D was enacted in 2003, the pharmaceutical companies were the beneficiaries of a huge financial windfall. Three legislators played a key role in the development of Medicare Part D. After Part D was enacted, congressman Billy Tauzin, Senators John Breaux and Don Nickles subsequently left government service and went to work for lobbying firms of the pharmaceutical companies. These firms paid them much larger salaries than they ever received as legislators. Billy Tauzin was hired by the biggest pharmaceutical lobby group known as PHARMA. His compensation was reported to be more than $2 million per year. ProPublica, the nonprofit journalism group, reported that twenty-seven former members of Congress, who were very influential in the design of Medicare Part D, went to work for the pharmaceutical companies regarding health-care reform. Not only are lobbyist organizations spending millions and millions of dollars to influence elections and enact legislation, they gain even more influence by paying outrageous salaries to those same legislators when they leave government service.

In health care overall, 267 former aides and 18 former lawmakers are registered lobbyists for the health-care sector and the health insurance industry. These former aides and lawmakers worked for committees that were key participants in the development of health-care legislation.

Litigation and Taxes

Litigations and abuses, both requiring huge attorney fees, have been a common occurrence in the industry. These costs are just another factor that are included in the premiums we pay.

Between August 9 and August 11, 2017, BC/BS of Michigan was sued more than thirty times by employers claiming the insurer skimmed unauthorized fees from their health-care plans. The lawsuits maintain that Blue Cross/Blue Shield charged hidden and unauthorized fees as part of their premiums for the sole purpose of improving their profits. The basis of the lawsuit was a 2014 appeals court decision that upheld that Blue Cross/Blue Shield was in violation of the Employee Retirement Income Security Act (ERISA) and had to pay the $6 million judgment that accompanied the suit. Following the court case more than two hundred employers claiming ERISA violations relating to hidden charges have filed suit against Blue Cross/Blue Shield.

In October 2016, a federal class action suit was filed against the insurer United Health Care. The suit claims that United Health Care, unbeknownst to its customers, overcharged them for prescription drugs. In one instance, a customer was overcharged $15.00 for a thyroid medication. In looking at her past purchase of the drug before she obtained coverage, she discovered she bought the drug cheaper prior to using her insurance.

In another example, Valsartan HCTZ, a high blood pressure medication, cost $14.43 if purchased without insurance. In using their insurance, the client was charged a $30 co-pay. The pharmacist kept $14.43 and reimbursed United Health Care $15.57. In the industry, this is referred to as a claw back.

Pharmacists across the country have cited other numerous examples including a $22.00 claw back on the nasal spray, Fluticasone, $7.85 for a diabetes treatment, Invokamet, and $12.39 for Diazepam, a drug that treats anxiety, muscle spasms, and seizures. In another extreme case, the patient paid $150 for a drug, but the pharmacist didn't get to keep the $150. The insurer clawed back $140.00 of the cost.

More than one expert in the industry have deemed the practice to be fraudulent and a misrepresentation to the paying consumer. United Health Care customers in New York, New Jersey, and Michigan have ongoing suits in federal court.

Blue Cross/Blue Shield is currently involved in an antitrust lawsuit alleging that the independently owned companies within the BCBS organization operate as an illegal cartel that controls premium pricing and provider reimbursements. Blue Cross/

LARRY STONE

Blue Shield companies cover about a third of all Americans. In some states like Mississippi, they cover 85 percent of the insured population, and in Alabama they cover 97 percent.

Prescription Drugs

One of the most heated health-care topics is the cost of prescription drugs in the United States. American consumers are constantly asking why the pharmaceutical companies charge so much for their medications. Without trying to be coy, it's because they can.

There are many different factors involved in the pricing of medications. Some are very legitimate. The cost of research, getting a drug approved, and bringing it to the marketplace are all costly endeavors. However, further scrutiny of how medications are priced reveals many abuses and pitfalls in the system resulting in unnecessary high prices.

It is well known that the same medication in different parts of the world is significantly cheaper than in the United States. According to the International Federation of Health Plans, Americans pay two to six times more than the rest of the world for brand name prescription drugs.

Examples	U.S.	Netherlands	England	Canada
Nexium	$215	$23		
Gleevec (cancer drug)	$6,214	$52	$2,246	$1,141
Cymbalta (for depression)	$194		$46	
Humira (for rheumatoid arthritis)	$2,246		$1,102	

Most experts agree that the main reason other nations pay less for medications is due to their negotiating power. Most nations around the world have a single-payor health-care system and negotiate directly with manufacturers on drug pricing for their entire population.

In contrast, the United States doesn't regulate drug prices or have a single-payor system. More than one health-care professional has publicly agreed with Dr. Peter Bach, director of Memorial Sloan Kettering's Center for Health Policy and Outcomes, when he stated, "We have no rational system in the US for managing the price of drugs." Drug manufacturers have demonstrated that they will use their powerful influences to enact favorable legislation that boosts profits or lobby against any changes that will adversely affect their bottom line. A classic example is Medicare, the largest provider of prescription drugs. Due to the successful efforts of the pharmaceutical lobby, they are forbidden, by law, to directly negotiate with drug manufacturers on pricing. It seems very ironic that the large pharmaceutical firms are proponents of less regulation in the free marketplace, but when it comes to protecting or increasing their profits, they sing a different song.

The Veterans Administration is a case in point on how regulations affect drug pricing. The VA is a completely self-contained health-care system and has for years negotiated directly with drug manufacturers. As a result, they save upward of 20 percent per medication compared to Medicare.

In the United States, each health-related entity, primarily health insurance companies, must individually negotiate with the pharmaceutical companies, resulting in higher drug prices. To curb costs, the health insurance industry in the United States uses highly controversial pharmacy benefit managers, known as PBMs, to negotiate drug pricing for their plans. PBMs maintain their actions result in lower pricing for the consumer. Although their claim has some validity, they also rake off a large part of any savings to create substantial profits.

A large percentage of Americans are unaware of how pharmacy benefit managers (PBMs) function. These large companies act as gatekeepers between your health plan and the drug companies. The three largest PBMs are Express Scripts, CVS Caremark, and Optimum United Health. These three companies control over 70 percent of the United States market. They negotiate directly with the pharmaceutical manufacturers for the lowest possible pricing, and these discounts are then marketed to health insurance companies including Medicaid providers. Again, another middleman integrated into our health-care system.

A classic example of anti-consumerism is the state of Ohio Medicaid program. PBM contracts for Medicaid with the state forbid the pharmacy from informing the patient when the prescription would be cheaper if they paid for their medication out of pocket. Legislators are appealing to the state attorney general to determine if this contract provision is legal. How these contracts were even approved in the first place is a question all Ohioans should be asking. Dr. Donald Wharton, Ohio Medicaid's assistant medical director, is beginning an analysis of what they pay managed care companies providing services to Medicaid recipients, what these companies pay the PBMs, and what the PBMs pay the pharmacies.

In a follow up article in the Columbus Dispatch on February 10, 2019, Governor Mike DeWine again accused the contracted PBMs of ripping–off Ohio tax payers of $224 million dollars through a loop hole that allowed them to charge a 10% mark up on what they paid the dispensing pharmacists. Antonio Ciaccia stated in the article that the PBMs contracts are complex by design thus giving the PBMs hidden streams of revenue which went undetected.

PBM companies like Express Scripts and CVS's Caremark have very little transparency and little regulation. To better understand their influence, Express Scripts is in the top 25 of American corporations, making it bigger than Microsoft. These companies are growing larger through mergers and acquisitions that will further subject the consumer to higher prices for their medications. As of this writing, CVS is looking to purchase Aetna for $68 billion. This will give CVS Caremark control of the insurance plan, the pharmacy, and the PBM. Through their vertical integration, the parent company would now have three separate profit centers. Independent pharmacists in Ohio and Arkansas have claimed that CVS Caremark reimburses their company owned pharmacies at a higher rate than the independent pharmacies they have under contract. Another health insurer, Cigna is attempting to purchase Express Scripts, the largest PBM in the United States for $54 billion. In the event these business deals take place, even more competition will be eliminated. Are we truly to believe that the elimination of competition will lower the cost of prescription drugs?

One horrific example and featured on CBS *60 Minutes* May 6, 2018, Express Scripts contracted with the city of Rockford, Illinois, to negotiate lower drug prices for their employee's health insurance. The drug Acthar, a treatment for a rare disease in children, was $40 a vial in 2002, and the city was charged $40,000 a vial. The manufacturer Questcor, a subsidiary of Mallinckrodt Pharmaceuticals, recently settled with the Federal Trade Commission for $100 million for violating antitrust laws regarding the drug. It is interesting to note, executive compensation at Mallinckrodt was $13.26 million in 2013 and soared to $41.79 million in 2017. As of this printing,

Express Scripts is also being sued for failing to negotiate for their client.

House Representative Doug Collins (R-GA), a member of House Speaker Ryan's leadership team, tactfully stated, "In light of the chronic mischief that PBMs create at the expense of patients and the community pharmacies that serve them, we continue to be concerned about the impact of consolidation in the health-care industry on market concentration and competition."

House Representative Earl "Buddy" Carter (R-GA), the only pharmacist in congress, was even more blunt and to the point. He stated, "Ask the PBMs what their mission is, they will tell you, we help keep drug prices low. Well, how is that working out?" He continued, "We know when CVS Caremark buys Aetna, they'll control the PBM, the insurance company, and the mail order pharmacy. What is going to happen is that you're going to have less competition and less choices for patients. When there is less competition, that means prices are going up and that's what is going to happen when we have this vertical integration."

Many physicians also contribute to the high-cost drugs. Large pharmaceutical companies financially reward physicians for endorsing and prescribing their drugs. This is especially prevalent in the very expensive medications.

If this all sounds very confusing, you are not alone. The industry by design is confusing, making it very difficult for the average American to get a clear understanding of the reasons for our health-care crisis. Quite frankly, I am unsure if our legislators comprehend all the issues.

Potential Solutions

Here comes the difficult part of the equation. Developing an alternative health-care system to what now exists will be a difficult task as our current system is so ingrained in our culture and business environment. With that said, unless changes or alternatives are put in place, we are headed for a crisis of significant proportions.

There exists a huge disagreement on whether we should have a national health-care plan that is funded by the US government for every citizen or for each citizen to be personally responsible for the cost. Whatever your viewpoint, neither one is feasible under the current system. Before we have that debate, we first need to enact reforms and make innovative changes that would make either way of providing health care more practical and cost effective.

Despite the many misconstrued myths, the Affordable Care Act (ACA) was a noble attempt for the masses to have access to health care. However, since its inception, costs have increased at such an alarming rate that many Americans cannot afford to purchase coverage, and this number will continue to rise.

THE AMERICAN HEALTH CARE CRISIS

Prior to the ACA, insurance carriers could deny coverage based on preexisting conditions. The enactment of the ACA required that all insurance carriers must accept all applicants regardless of health conditions. As costs continued to rise, low risk insured elected not to purchase coverage. Consequently, too large of a percentage of the individuals enrolled were high risk patients. For any pool of insured to remain solvent, it must be composed of both high and low risk individuals to create an equal balance between claims and premiums.

The core problem with the ACA is that the insurance companies in the plan are primarily for-profit businesses with their main concern of maximizing profits. Concerns of providing low cost and affordable health insurance is the least of their objectives. Many members of congress claim that the ACA needs to offer additional plans that have less benefits and would be cheaper for the consumer. While this could very well be true and perhaps be a good option, it doesn't solve the problem. You are still going to pay too high a cost for whatever benefit level you choose. With this concept, you will pay less in monthly premiums, but you will pay higher co-pays for office visits and have higher deductibles.

The cost of quality health care will always be a significant expense, but the cost doesn't have to break the bank. Even in a true nonprofit plan, costs will rise due to Americans living longer, ever changing advances in medicine and rising salaries for those involved in the medical profession. In a nonprofit plan, these cost factors will be much more manageable as they will be more in line with inflation factors of our economy.

In the past few years, the way we deliver health care in our society has undergone some major changes that could potentially lead to other very viable alternatives. Hospitals in the past few years have gone into a merger mode. Large hospitals have joined with other large hospitals to form complete healthcare delivery networks. The majority of physicians have left private practice to become an integral part of these health-care delivery systems.

Keeping in mind the beginnings of health insurance, let's look at another scenario. Let us eliminate the traditional carrier with all their excessive costs and contract directly with the hospital. With no middlemen and no profits, the hospital would receive only the needed revenue to cover the cost of providing care. Remember why health care for the uninsured was initially designed?

Direct contracting would drastically reduce the cost of processing claims. Hospitals and insurance carriers openly admit that claim processing is a huge expense. Hospitals must employ a huge staff for filing claims, disputing claims, and following up on unpaid claims. Insurance companies have the burden of verifying claims, verifying eligibility, and processing payments. Reducing claim processing costs is another factor that would lower the cost of health care.

Most Americans are unaware that direct contracting is already taking place in the marketplace.

THE AMERICAN HEALTH CARE CRISIS

Direct marketing has been so far limited to employer groups providing health-care benefits to their employees. This method of providing health care has proven to drastically lower costs and have a huge impact on stabilizing future costs. The well-known technology company Intel implemented a direct contracting arrangement with eight hospitals and one hundred clinics across the state of Texas. They expect to show a savings of $8 to $10 million through 2017. A small company of two hundred employees in Indiana realized a savings of 50 percent between 2011 and 2012. In 2018, Reuters reported that some of America's largest corporations are exploring abandoning the middleman and insurers involved with their healthcare plan and contracting directly with providers of medical services.

Savings will vary depending on the type and level of benefits for which employers elect to direct contract. Of the small number of employers who have elected to direct contract for their benefits, some have chosen to only direct contract for such serious illnesses as cancer and cardiac issues. These health conditions result in very high claims and can quickly drive up employer premiums. One thing is for certain, by eliminating the for-profit insurance carrier and directly contracting with providers of health care, costs are lowered.

Many Americans believe they should be able to choose any health-care provider for their medical needs. Unfortunately, this is an option that is very expensive. Plans must be able to negotiate discounts with providers by promising large volumes of business to keep their premiums as low as possible. There are very few plans available today that allow you to choose your physician or hospital. However, the plans that offer you that choice are very expensive.

Direct contracting by employers is a cost-effective way of controlling benefit costs. Most employers will readily admit that the cost of health benefits for their employees is second only to wages. But in recent years, fewer and fewer employers are not even electing to provide or offer benefits to their employees due to high costs. Industries such as the hospitality sector have traditionally never offered benefits. That, combined with a huge portion of our economy consisting of very small businesses and self-employed individuals, means millions of Americans are left out in the cold when it comes to obtaining health care.

A hospital in the Midwest is a good example of an alternative way of delivering health-care. Their comprehensive health-care delivery system has a well-known cardiology department, a leading cancer center, general family practitioners, and other capabilities to deliver all forms of health care. Why can't this provider offer a plan that is available to everyone in the community? If most uninsured Americans are asked why they don't have health care, they will quickly reply that coverage is something they just can't afford. An affordable, nonprofit community-based plan would be an option for all these individuals and also a great option for those looking to reduce their current health-care premiums.

THE AMERICAN HEALTH CARE CRISIS

Once the pool of individuals participating in the plan grows, providers would not be forced to write off the large amount of medical bills incurred by those individuals who do not have the ability to pay. Eliminating the majority of these losses would enable large organizations to charge less for their services.

As it pertains to pharmaceutical companies and the high cost of prescription drugs, multiple options are at our disposal. As one example, hospitals would purchase needed drugs through their own pharmacies at wholesale pricing with maybe a small administration fee for dispensing. Regulations need to be enacted to regulate pricing. The wholesale cost of a drug in a foreign country should be the same price in the United States. Basically, the American consumer is subsidizing the drug industry's profits by allowing those companies to sell their drugs at a lesser cost to other nations around the world. We could develop a national pricing board that could be part of the Food and Drug Administration

The issues do offer some complex problems although not as complex as the industry and our legislators lead you to believe. What happens when someone is traveling overseas or domestically and needs medical attention? Here is where the traditional insurance companies come into play. Consumers could purchase a supplemental plan that only would be effective when they travel. These types of policies could be offered for many different levels of coverage from basic to catastrophic care.

Remember, insurance is just a pool of money designed to allow for risk and avoid financial catastrophes. More affordable coverage would motivate more individuals to enroll. As enrollment grows, risk continues to be spread out further lowering costs. With today's technology, why shouldn't we let the hospital handle the money? As previously illustrated, the pioneers of health-care insurance quickly realized that this was the most efficient and low-cost way to get health care to the masses. The system worked very well until big business got involved.

A CALL TO ACTION

MOST OF US ARE CONCERNED about the quality of life for our children and grandchildren. The current health-care crisis is only going to get worse, and unless we act, our future generations of Americans will face a crisis of tremendous proportions.

The health insurance and pharmaceutical companies are spending hundreds of millions of dollars in lobbying and political contributions to sway our politicians to enact favorable legislation to increase their net income. As citizens, it's time to start demanding that our elected officials separate themselves from the influence of the health-care industry and start enacting true reforms that will benefit all Americans.

Regardless of your position on gun control, the movement by our nation's students to enact gun reform demonstrates that we have the power to draw attention to a particular issue and bring about change.

Through new technology and the internet, we have many tools at our disposal. The website OpenSecrets.org has amassed readily available, public information on the voting record of our legislators for all to see. By searching the internet, we can learn how legislators are voting on certain bills and who is contributing to their campaigns. Never in our history has the American voter had access to so much information. Every legislator has a website and an e-mail address where we can communicate our views and opinions.

Have your congressman put you on his e-mail list and to inform you on how he voted on all health-care-related legislation. Don't just e-mail him or her once but do it on a regular basis. Invite them to a town hall meeting in your neighborhood. When we begin to make our legislators more accountable, things will change.

Some would argue, and I would probably agree, that the legislative branch of our government does not always properly serve its constituents. But we all have a vote, and we need to make ourselves heard at the polls. This is the greatest country in the world, and we can accomplish anything to which we apply our collective, informed efforts.

Refer to these websites for the legislator that represents your district or state: *www.senate.gov*

www.house.gov

We can all start the process by asking some very basic questions:

Why are the health insurance and pharmaceutical companies spending so much money lobbying to influence our lawmakers?

How much money did your campaign receive in political contributions from the health insurance and pharmaceutical lobby?

THE AMERICAN HEALTH CARE CRISIS

Why do we have a law that doesn't allow Medicare, the largest purchaser of prescription drugs, to negotiate drug prices directly with the manufacturers, and what are you doing to repeal that legislation?

Why can't we enact legislation that demands that the pharmaceutical companies sell their products at the same price to American consumers that they sell to other nations?

How do you plan on reducing health-care costs?

What are you doing to develop true nonprofit, community-based plans or other alternatives?

What is your position on the current activity of mergers in the health-care industry?

What is your stance on PBMs?

Consequences of Change

The health-care industry is a huge sector of our GDP, and any significant reduction in costs will have a positive ripple effect throughout the economy. Let us not debate liberal or conservative views as both sides of the aisle have legitimate arguments. Those on the right are of the opinion that the government cannot be part of a national health-care plan as it will drive the country farther into the already out-of-control national debt. Those on the left maintain that health care is the right of every American. Certainly, at a minimum, both parties would or should agree that affordable health insurance should be a number one priority.

The average American family spends upwards of 25 percent of their income on health care. Taking an annual income of $50,000 with $12,500 spent on health care, cutting health care costs by 40 percent would result in $5,000 of additional disposable income annually. One can only surmise what a boost this would be to our economy. Statistics show that as a nation, we now spend more money per capita on health care than any other country in the world.

For those whose primary concern is the huge portion of the federal budget being spent on entitlement programs, lower health-care costs would significantly reduce the amount of money dedicated to those programs. Think about all the employers who would see a reduction in their health-care costs and how those dollars could be spent in higher wages and improvements in their lines of business.

Just reforming the multibillion-dollar pharmaceutical industry could produce immediate positive results for every American. State governments and the federal government could lower entitlement costs and still provide benefits under Medicare and Medicaid. As discussed earlier, just letting Medicare negotiate drug prices, like the VA, could result in a minimum savings of 20 percent.

We all need to come together to fix a health-care system that is broken. The current system is an albatross around the neck of our federal budget, every state budget, every business, and every American.

REFERENCES AND CREDITS

Becker Hospital Review (www.beckerhospitalreview.com)
Bloomberg Law / Jacklyn Willie (www.bna.com)
Business Wire (www.businesswire.com)
CBS News / Sharyl Attkisson (www.cbsnews.com)
Center for Responsive Politics (www.opensecrets.org)
Columbus Dispatch / Catherine Candisky and Darrel Rowland (www.dispatch.com)
Fox 8 / Lee Zurik (www.fox8live.com)
Huffington Post / Sarah Bryner (www.huffingtonpost.com)
MarketWatch (www.marketwatch.com)
Morningstar (www.morningstar.com)
NASDQ (www.nasdq.com)
Nation, The / Michelle Chen (www.thenation.com)
New York Times / Milt Freudenheim (www.nytimes.com)
Propublica (www.propublica.org)
The Blues: History of the Blue Cross and Blue Shield System, by Robert Cunningham Jr. and Robert Cunningham III *USA Today* / Jayne O'Donnell (www.usatoday.com)
U.S. Securities and Exchange (www.sec/gov)

About the Author

Larry Stone spent years in the insurance industry. During his career, he often negotiated with medical providers and medical organizations to reduce their usual and customary fees. He founded Total Vision Services which negotiated directly with optical providers of vision care to offer vision benefits to employer groups. He was featured and recognized in the Cincinnati Business Currier as an innovative entrepreneur in the employee benefit market. Since his retirement, he has dedicated much of his time to educating the general public and talking to legislators about our healthcare crisis.